"I dressed his wounds, God healed him."
Ambroise Paré

"Science is one thing, wisdom is another."
Thomas Love Peacock

"The mere looking at externals is a matter for clowns, but the intuition of internals is a secret which belongs to physicians."
Paracelsus

"It is not possible to consider this as a medical side issue. Its permanence reflects an existing public need which is in urgent need of definition and analysis."
Council of Europe Report on the role of natural medicine in Europe, 1983

NOTE

As this monograph went to press (May 1986) the Report of the Board of Science Working Party on Alternative Therapy was published by the British Medical Association. Its general conclusions were that most of the therapies it examined were both ineffective and without scientific basis. It did however stress that the time given to their patients by many alternative practitioners was undoubtedly a potent factor in improving a suffer's response to his condition. The members of the Working Party are said to have had little or no experience of other therapies while, as the author suggests, their medical colleagues who have would often strongly disagree with their conclusions, except no doubt the last.

The BMA is of course committed to scientific validation and rightly so. However, and again the author makes this point, alternative or complementary practice frequently insists that current methods of scientific investigation are either insufficently sensitive to uncover the basis on which it works; or that this is actually outside the scope of science as at present understood.

The Healing Within
Medicine, Health and Wholeness

A generational transaction

We have come a long way since Stewart Brand looked down from his California-bound jet and conceived the idea of the *Whole Earth Catalog*. Based on the understanding that the world is one, it listed in Sears and Roebuck manner all kinds of things pertaining to the alternative lifestyle from the Abacus to Zen. It included organic farming, intermediate technology, flower power, solar heating, and much else from the sane to the zany. Itself a product of an uncommon concern, it triggered thought and activity on a far wider scale than its modest newsprint appearance would have suggested.

How far have we come since those heady days of the 1960s? Medicine, as a precise indicator of the society which gives it rise, changes constantly, both in the limited sense of conventional, National Health Service medicine, and in its complementary associates. It may be useful to tease out the present state of official medicine and of complementary medicine in order to see what may, or may not, associate the two.

Official medicine in the United Kingdom is of course a huge national enterprise. It employs many people, spent in 1983-84 some £15,700m, and in the last year for which figures are available dealt with 6.180m in-patients and 37m out-patients; both figures are up on the previous year. A service with diminishing real funds and decreasing staff which provides such support is not doing at all badly. It owns vast and enormously complex and expensive hospitals whose equipment is capital-intensive and expensive to maintain. Its medical and nursing staff is highly-trained and highly motivated. Its general practitioners, as front-line troops in the battle against ill-health, are usually the first recourse of patients; where the practitioner thinks it necessary the patient will be passed to specialists in hospitals for fuller treatment. We all have cause to be immensely grateful both for ourselves and for others for the safety-net which this service represents.

And yet much is wrong, not only with the dire effects of much of the treatment, but also with the muddled and inadequate philosophy which lies behind its practice. Effects of the one we can all probably quote from our own experience, that of friends, or from casual newspaper reading: treatment of the wrong lung for pneumonia, amputations of the wrong limb, maintenance of life support systems when the patient is in any meaningful sense long since dead. Or, devotion in the past to such fashionable and frequently unnecessary surgical interventions as appendectomy, tonsillectomy, removal of the gall bladder, and until recently to hyper-medication by tranquillisers. Or, the lavish application of the latest cure-all: penicillin and cortisone, marvellously effective in controlled use, are demonic in effect when used without discretion. Chemotherapy for cancer is notoriously uncertain in therapeutic value. We do know, however, that its side effects may well, and often do, outweigh its therapeutic effects. We tend to forget that the side-effect is, in fact, the effect.

Surgical intervention and medical therapeutics are one thing; diagnostics are another. Patients, particularly those who are ignorant or inarticulate, may be subjected to diagnostic processes whose value is somewhat questionable, and whose effect could be to bring about the death of the patient: cardiac catheterisation is a dangerous and some would say still an experimental process. It is noticeable that the dangers of such procedures are often only vouchsafed on the patient's request. Safer diagnostics, for instance X-ray examination of the digestive system, are carried out efficiently, promptly and with due precaution; they are, nevertheless, carried out without any consideration for the patient as a sentient and territorial being. He is stripped of his clothes, put in a standard hospital gown, sat among others equally unidentifiable on a row of upright chairs around a bare room and he waits until his number is called (significant phrase). Strapped to a vast and moving table, he is later ejected with disfavour and discovers for himself much later that the barium meal still clings to his lips. Comic, yes; but strangely dislocated as a medical procedure. So also the surprise with which medical staff continue to note that the blind often cannot voluntarily move their eyes when asked to do so for diagnostic and therapeutic purposes. Appalling hospital food, processed, overcooked, unappetising, if indeed not unavailable through staff strikes, is another area fit for radical improvement: it is disgraceful that patients are not given the nutrition that they need for recovery. The high expenditure, high technology, labour-intensive, symptomatic aspects of conventional hospital factory-medicine symbolise very precisely an unthinking attachment to the technological utopianism of the post-war years.

The engineering 'pill for every ill', oppositional 'battle-front' form of medicine is often repeated at general practitioner level, where depersonalisation is carried, often through no immediate fault of the practitioner, to extremes. The practitioner, tired, harried, overloaded with cases, sometimes of up to 60 in an evening, cannot be blamed if he treats each patient as a two-minute 'encapsulated case', provides a quick therapeutic piece of paper and so fulfils and reinforces his and his patient's assumption that medicine is a commodity for rapid exchange.

The upshot of this and of hospital medicine, is that, according to different assessments, from 5 per cent to 18 per cent of all hospital cases are iatrogenic, that is, medically induced: a tale of human woe which should never be. Horror stories abound: but let it suffice, that many excesses are beginning to be recognised by an increasingly critical clientèle. Tranquillisers for example are on the way out: *Tranx*, an organisation dedicated to weaning patients from them, has produced a book ingeniously entitled *Bottling it up*, a title which says much in brief of the unwritten agenda of conventional medicine.

None of this is exaggerated: every detail is perfectly true. Many of us can produce worse and more painful stories. While Ivan Illich's splendid paradox that 'the medical establishment has become a major threat to health' goes much too far in vilification, we can surely repeat with Sir Robert Hutchison his new petition for the Anglican Litany:

> "From inability to let well alone; from too much zeal for the new and contempt for what is old; from putting knowledge before wisdom; science before art, and cleverness before common sense, from treating patients as cases, and from making the cure of the disease more grievous than the endurance of the same, Good Lord deliver us."

It must also be said that there are and always have been many practitioners within the hospitals who are able, courteous, and sensitive, and who have in fact done much to mitigate the factory style of conventional medicine. Of them and of new and happier developments within the area of received medicine, more later.

Form, structure, hierarchy, vested interest, the coercive power of a religion vested in scientific positivism, a profound theological inertia has prevented the acceptance of ideas outside the familiar formulae of yet bigger and more complex technology.

The problem may lie in the assumption that treating the presenting ill is the whole nature of medicine. The assumption is antique, respectable, and obvious. It is also charitable, and it merits our respect. In spite of its many mis-aims, no one would deny that the medical profession cares about its patients and that within its conceptual, practical and economic limitations it does its best for them. Its many specialities perform wonders; and conditions which a generation ago would have been considered hopeless are now routinely treated and cured.

Some say that the dislocation of medicine lies in the divorce between curing and caring; and this to some extent must be so. A piece of paper delivered at speed is no substitute for the listening authority figure, a fact which is increasingly recognised if, owing to the same shortage of time, little acted upon. But the major dislocation may lie in the profession's unwillingness and inability to promote health, in the sense of steering the potential patient away from the manifestation of disease long before he gets there. This reluctance may itself be a product of an uncertainty as to the nature of health, and what patterns such a condition represents. Such a search by medicine for the knowledge it lacks may discover a subtler understanding of energy relationships within the body-spirit continuum whose balance is vital to the harmony of the individual. Such energy relationships are already to some extent recognised by the profession as the basis of acupuncture therapy. If such relationships exist, presenting symptoms may then be regarded, more wholly and usefully, as the broken lights of a greater harmony. If we pass, as this concept suggests, from the simple to the complex, from the subtle to the coarse, it should not be a matter for surprise that we discover confusion of aims, apparently irreconcilable opposites, dissatisfactions, and a search for more appropriate therapies.

Given the oppositional assumptions of most of us, it is obvious that an alternative schema to the inadequacies of conventional medicine would be presented. The opposition is in fact most recognisably reflected in the Alternative Medicine Exhibition held for the past four years in Kensington: it is a showcase for all alternative therapies and for the institutions associated with them. In 1985 some 14,000 visitors attended during the four days of the exhibition. The same year saw over 170 stands ranging from materials on the Alexander Technique to Zodiac Gems. Superficially, the hardsell counts, and much *is* sold, from Bach Flower Remedies to alternative seating systems and Aurora crystals; but there are quieter stalls, where the purveyors of remedies, the interpreters of therapeutic systems, and contact and distant healers may be met. Demonstrations and lectures are held, and the atmosphere is one of a market where ideas, apparatus, systems, and therapeutic substances are discussed and exchanged. Seen from the outside, it is lively, eccentric, sometimes absurd, often amusing and entertaining. It is above all alive and stimulating.

What does this freewheeling and cheerful exterior represent? Briefly, most practitioners in these apparently diverse fields would claim that the body heals itself if given the opportunity; that the underlying cause of a disease must be identified and treated; that since we operate at the multi-dimensional levels of mind, emotion and spirit, a balance between them must be found; that the spirit is the source and centre of our healing; and because this is so, the patient as a whole person must be part of the healing process. Every patient is unique. There is no one treatment in its standard form which is right for all patients. The Alexander Technique, for instance, depends for its efficacy on the participation of the patient; while for another patient the stronger and more interventionist approach of Ortho-bionomy would be more effective. For another, perhaps, reflexology would provide the return to balance and the means to growth.

In the best circumstances therefore the healer is the catalyst for better understanding on the part of the patient, for his release from the misunderstanding that had chained him, into a renewed possibility for growth. As one practitioner puts it: "The patient is not a victim; he must have the energy and inner direction to heal; the patient is the Managing Director in the process; he is in charge; he takes responsibility. The aim of the treatment is to return the patient to a state of potency within his realm."

The means of carrying out this programme are as diverse as the whole spectrum of alternative medicine. They will range from dietary reform, particularly among those who claim that processed and sprayed food are responsible for much sub-clinical ill health, to contact (spiritual) healing, to distant healing (spiritual healing and radionics), to such symptomatic therapies as homoeopathy and the use of the vital essence of flowers, to such physical approaches as acupuncture, naturopathy, osteopathy and chiropractic, or the latest and most trumpeted natural remedy. In fact, from the outer environment to the inner environment of the patient, from his coarser to his finer substances. Some practitioners would claim that the body is a temporary phenomenon and that it is best understood as a metaphor of a spiritual mode of being. The full curative aim, therefore, lies beyond physical health. Illness becomes thus a crisis which the therapist is there to help the patient to solve. Therapists speak of the power of unconditional acceptance — or unaffective love — as the transpersonal resolution of the distress their patients suffer and which has translated itself into disease.

Most people are now aware in crude but sufficient terms of the aims and means of the major methods of alternative medicine. A few comments on some of them will therefore suffice to place the reader within the picture. The environmental field is covered in part by the whole food movement, a descendant of the Whole Earthism of the 1960s, and more critically by the new interest in clinical ecology. The latter concerns itself with the interaction between the human organism and its environment, paying particular attention to the allergic reactions and chemical intolerances which, it is claimed, are increasingly provoked by the methods of the food-processing business, of agriculture and of industry in general. The clinical ecologists see in these methods the roots of much of the persistent low-grade ill health which fills doctors' surgeries all over the world and which often seems to defy conventional treatment. In another sphere, spiritual healing is now regularly taught to those capable of receiving it; such healers are said to number some 20,000 in the United Kingdom alone.

Homoeopathy, a symptomatic system, believes that 'like cures like' and doses its patients on amounts so minute of the substance which produces the symptoms that the practitioners seek to remedy, that the therapeutic substance cannot in any material sense be said still to exist. Nevertheless, 'succussed' and therefore potentiated, the remedies are claimed to be highly effective and entirely safe when prescribed by an experienced practitioner. High potencies and over-dosing are to be avoided by the uninformed. There is great emphasis in homoeopathic practice on matching the remedy to the patient. Cases which are apparently identical may receive quite different treatments.

Radionics, a system of distant diagnostics and healing, has affinities with both homoeopathy and with the vital essences of flowers and gems whose remedial patterns it often seeks to transmit to its patients. Broadly, it is both a means of diagnosis and a means of cure. The diagnosis may be arrived at by means of a pendulum operated by a sensitive and skilled practitioner, who having diagnosed the dis-ease (often one whose source would never be suspected by the conventional system), sets up on the dials of his so-called 'black box' the appropriate remedy rate for the therapeutic substance he broadcasts to the patient. He may simply broadcast the appropriate rate or a 'pattern of health' arrived at by intuition and knowledge. A practitioner may also require the patient to undertake other treatments whether physical or homoeopathic. The aim is to restore as full a condition of balance and harmony as possible.

In parenthesis, implications of the radionic principle that the body is a series of harmonies in which dis-harmony is related to dis-ease has led to the possibility that the wrong harmony may be displaced by the harmony appropriate to the affected organ. A practitioner in this advanced field has pointed out that the human body is analogous to a symphony; though every cell is essentially the same, each has its particular function and operates within its own organic system at an optimum harmonic rate. A machine now exists which is said to implant into the misdirected structure the corrected harmonic frequency. By correcting the signal and feeding it back into the affected organ, the machine, it is claimed, can stabilise cases and even reverse them. Cases involving unalleviated pain, patients wearing pacemakers, and psychopathic cases are not appropriate for this treatment; however, arthritis, stress and tension are said to answer well; also cases of drug addiction, since the drug in question may be safely emulated by frequency and so gradually diminished. It is obvious that if this system is viable, the exchange of one frequency for another may have profound implications for the treatment of certain cancers; this assumption remains to be tested.

Herbalism, as the oldest of all therapies, enjoys a particular esteem in the United Kingdom, partly because it is recognisably if deceptively similar to the conventional medicine which in fact grew out of it. The actual resemblance is not that great, since the herbal practitioner again claims that the set parameters of medicine are totally inappropriate. In the herbal system the one condition, apparently the same in two patients, may call for two entirely different remedies. Rather as in homoeopathy, each condition is unique to the patient, and each medicine is unique to its recipient. The purpose of herbal therapy is to identify the problem and to raise the body's ability to heal itself.

Osteopathy, which seeks to correct malfunctions of the musculoskeletal system, is by now familiar to many people. It is sometimes identified with chiropractic, but this, although also manipulative, tends to concentrate on disorders of the spine. The Alexander Technique concerns itself with postural re-education as a means to health and is another of the physical approaches to whole treatment. Among these we might also include acupuncture which works on the principle that the organs of the body are linked by energetic pathways (whose nature is as yet unknown) to certain points on or near the body's surface. By inserting one or more needles at an appropriate point, the flow of energy can be affected and a specific organ stimulated to repair itself. A related idea underlies reflexology, except that here reflexes linked to all parts of the body are located in the feet or hands and stimulation is produced by pressure applied to the reflex points. The factor common to all these methods is that they all seek to identify points of crisis in the patient, to bring the physical manifestation back into balance and to restore the free flow of energy. Their techniques are of course very different, and the treatment that will be effective for one patient will be less effective for another. Here, as elsewhere, it is for the patient as well as the therapist to establish the appropriate treatment.

Given the oppositional elements implicit in the conventional and alternative attitudes towards health and healing it is not surprising that experiments in compromise are being made. A pivotal enterprise is the Bristol Cancer Help Centre, set up in 1980, which has now grown into new premises, has borrowed a large sum of money to enable it to do so, and whose staff is headed by a team of qualified registered medical practitioners. Patients attend daily, for a week or two, or for longer. They come from the United Kingdom and from every continent. The treatment, which looks at the whole patient — the body, mind and spirit — aims at the cause rather than the effect. Its treatments can safely be used alongside orthodox treatments; and they are intended to complement and enhance orthodox effectiveness. Patients are taught the importance of what they eat (a recent study in the USA has shown that 35 per cent of cancers were caused by the wrong foods); they are helped to discover the cause of their originating stress and how to handle it; and they are offered contact healing. A wholefood, largely vegetarian and raw food diet is provided, and medical counselling, personal counselling, and relaxation are offered. Patients are given the opportunity to come to terms with their condition, to release emotional burdens, to build up more positive attitudes and to live in harmony with themselves and their environment.

Placing the patient within his background of cultural expectation has been the theme of medical anthropology. While perhaps superficially more pedestrian and intellectual than other means of understanding, it does in fact seek to recognise the sets of assumptions ('Chinese boxes') within which both medical practitioner and patient live. It seeks, by understanding these unwritten cultural commitments, to make the curative process more immediate and more complete. The concept of medical anthropology is now well understood and, indeed, institutionalised in the USA; while in the UK it is accepted in some medical schools and in the instruction of general practitioners as part of their educational programme.

Other less identifiable moves have been made within conventional areas of medicine within recent years. The introduction of bran and wholefood is in part the product of the Whole Earth movement, and it is now regarded by established medicine as scientifically sound for general nutrition as well as for the treatment of conditions as diverse as heart disease, varicose veins and diverticulitis. The addictive and personality-changing dangers of tranquillisers have been noted. Childbirth, while enjoying where necessary all the life-saving apparatus of hospitalisation, gives full place to the mother, child and the father: it is now not unusual for the father to be present at the birth. Massage is provided for cardiac patients at Charing Cross Hospital, London. Hypnotherapy is available at Leeds General Infirmary. The Great Ormond Street Hospital for Sick Children encourages parents to look after their children both when they are in the hospital and later at home. It is reported by medical staff that such parents become more expert in the specialised care of their sick children than the local hospitals. One medical commentator on this development has called attention to the way in which 'ordinary people become extraordinary'.

Most of us have heard of the elaborate health farms which make simple living, rest, exercise and a general regimen available to refugees from the urban race. Many will also have heard of the hospice movement, again supplementary to conventional medicine, which provides an accepting and controlled ambiance for the dying.

Transformation can take place here too. Staff often speak of their hospices as places of joy. Perhaps more unusual and less well known is the medical research programme to establish scientifically the efficacy of spiritual or contact healing. The project, which is expected to last from six months to two years, is taking place simultaneously in five medical centres around the UK. It will concentrate on five conditions: cataract, rheumatoid arthritis, cancer, pain (neuralgia and sprain) and a condition known as blue oedema for which there is said to be no medical treatment. Dr Alex Forbes, founder of the Bristol Cancer Help Centre, believes that on average healers have a 60 per cent rate of improving a patient's condition; occasionally 'a few miraculous cures' occur. Interestingly, and perhaps surprisingly, one healer claims that the most dramatic results are obtained with sufferers from multiple sclerosis.

Furthermore, the doctors themselves are taking an increasingly informed interest in alternative medicine. The interest is both institutional and individual. Some two years ago the British Medical Association set up its working party on alternative therapies. So far some 120 therapies are being investigated. The Royal Society of Medicine has allowed conferences on alternative medicine to take place within its premises. More radically, it has established a series of colloquia on orthodox and complementary medicine initiated by the Prince of Wales and attended by him. At such meetings the suspicions and prejudices on both sides of the medical fence are noticeably decreased and even harmonised. What is particularly interesting is that a number of senior members of the medical profession are deeply concerned with the state of their profession, with its limitations and with its mechanistic view of the human condition; so much so, that some have come to recognise that certain aspects of alternative medicine may indeed, as its practitioners prefer to claim, with appropriate safeguards, become recognised as complementary to conventional medicine.

Individual interest elsewhere in the profession remains high. The survey of general practitioners' attitudes to alternative medicine, conducted by *The Times* and the Koestler Foundation, using a nationally representative sample of 108 practitioners, made some surprising discoveries. A majority (57 per cent) would like to use alternative therapies. Those qualifying in 1970 and thereafter are the most interested: figures which are borne out by research on a group of 100 general practitioner trainees published in the *British Medical Journal* (30 July 1983), which demonstrated that 18 already used at least one alternative therapy, that 22 either had been treated or had treated themselves by means of an alternative therapy, and that 70 would like to have training in one or more of the therapies. *The Times* enquiry discovered that more than 50 per cent of those using or referring patients to acupuncture and osteopathy said that they were 'very or quite satisfied'; 18 of 34 were 'very or quite satisfied' with chiropractic; and 21 of 39 were similarly satisfied with meditation and relaxation.

With the growing interest in alternative medicine and positive health rather than the treatment of disease, the interest in beneficent lifestyles, and in attaining inner harmony, it is not surprising that the inherently fissiparous nature of the alternative medicine movement has excited comment both from within its ranks and from without. A movement whose means to the end of healing are apparently so varied and whose purposes are qualitative rather than quantitative cannot but be difficult to define to itself and to others. Conventional medicine, before it can treat with so diverse an object, will need a definitive exterior and a representative body with which it can negotiate. Demands have been made on both sides of the curtain for alternative medicine to put its house in order; demands which become more pressing with the report that more than 1m people in the UK each year choose alternative therapy treatment and that some 10m had consulted alternative practitioners by 1981.

Order is being discovered. At least two bodies presently exist: the Institute for Complementary Medicine (ICM) and the Council for Complementary and Alternative Medicine (CCAM). That there is more than one body at this stage should cause neither surprise nor grief. Live movements throw off energy like the sun. The first, a prestigious body, with offices in Portland Place, London, founded in 1981, aims to represent the movement at a senior level, to be a meeting-place for the official therapy bodies whose representatives form their educational and advisory committees, and to provide a much-needed computerised information centre open to the media, researchers and the general public. It has set up Public Information Points manned by volunteers who provide information to enquirers, public classes and lecturers, self-help and self-care, and discussions. Perhaps most usefully, it has placed alternative medicine and its problems of identification, examination, and authentication on the public stage by means of a two-hour debate in the House of Lords on 27 February 1985. The debate continued to urge, without seeking to adopt any one institution, greater order in the affairs of alternative medicine.

Curiously, on the previous day, Tuesday 26 February 1985, the CCAM was set up at the House of Commons at a meeting presided over by Lord Home of the Hirsel. It gained the support of an all-party group of MPs and, more importantly for its immediate future, it was founded after much preliminary background negotiation, with the full support of eight major professional alternative associations: the British Naturopathic and Osteopathic Association, the British Chiropractic Association, the College of Osteopaths, the National Institute of Medical Herbalists, the Society of Homoeopaths, the British Acupuncture Association, the Traditional Acupuncture Society, and the Register of Traditional Chinese Medicine. Between them they represent some 1,200 practising UK therapists. Two well-regarded osteopathic associations have refused to join on the grounds that they have no need to improve their standards of qualification; however, the chairman of the CCAM regards the eight organisations as foundation members to be added to as the occasion arises. He also makes the point that the Council's exercise is indeed both alternative and complementary — alternative in the sense that it applies alternative approaches but does not attack the medical establishment, complementary in the sense that it would prefer to work with the medical profession. There is a place for both the alternative and the complementary mode. As an umbrella organisation, intended by all participating bodies at the start as a co-ordinative enterprise to concentrate on producing a single register, common ethics, disciplinary procedures and a high standard of education, CCAM does have outstanding possibilities for success. It is fairly evident that both ICM and CCAM will need to bring their cohorts together in favour of one comprehensive body. Two separate registers are unlikely to be tolerated for long either by their own associates, by the medical profession, or by Government when it seeks to treat with alternative medicine as a body.

Two other organisations of prime significance have also been founded in the recent past, both in 1983. The British Holistic Medical Association (BHMA), a group of doctors and medical students, with the motto 'physician heal thyself', aims to introduce holistic medicine into contemporary medical practice. While continuing to make use of all appropriate therapies from orthodox medicine, it also seeks to recognise the uniqueness of the patient and his ability, with guidance and help, to treat himself. Health care, prevention and sometimes the cure can be brought about by seeking psychological, emotional and spiritual health. To this end it uses also alternative methods of treatment, and self-help skills such as breathing and relaxation routines, meditation, visualisation, physical exercise and dietary changes. The Positive Health Centre in London, run by one of its members, uses these techniques. BHMA's publications include the excellent *British Journal of Holistic Medicine* (soon to be re-published by a major publisher as *Holistic Medicine*) and its three-monthly useful and informative *Newsletter*. It has set up an Associate Membership open to the lay public and the British Association for Holistic Health for those in the National Health Service and others who work holistically with patients or clients to help them improve and maintain their health. Its conferences, workshops, lectures, and above all its existence within the medical profession is likely to have a remarkably powerful leavening influence on medical philosophy and practice.

The Research Council for Complementary Medicine (RCCM) is also at the centre of a major development in the alternative health field. An intelligent, careful, negotiatory, and catalytic enterprise, the RCCM has been set up to encourage the incorporation of the best in the alternative field into the mainstream of modern medical practice. In doing so it recognises the twin difficulties of poor information and poor methodological reporting. It has therefore stimulated funding for a part-time researcher to set up an Information Access Centre at the British School of Osteopathy; the British Library is associated with the project to ensure compatibility of systems and that effort is not duplicated. The RCCM, and the Medical Research Council — the association of the two is itself a significant step forward — have jointly funded a Research Methodology Fellowship to which an appointment has now been made. The RCCM is at pains to point out that it belongs to no one party within alternative medicine and that it seeks only to bring about greater understanding between conventional medicine and what it would prefer to call complementary medicine. It is obvious that a programme of such research in a field where conventional methodologies are by no means always appropriate must have a significant impact at a time when the British Medical Association is due to make its own report on alternative therapies. The existence of a median view at such a time is highly desirable, and one awaits with greatest interest the findings of the RCCM researcher in a field so extraordinary diverse.

Conclusions

The basic tenet of holistic medicine is that the best healing is self-help and self-healing. It is something you do rather than have done to you. It seeks to educe individuated, self-motivated beings. As products of a distorted and mechanical society, this is precisely the medicine that is needed to redress the balance in the individual and in society. It allows passage to the *vis medicatrix naturae* — 'the healing force of nature' — it expects the individual to make his own decisions and to take responsibility for them. It is essentially anti-statist, anti-bureaucratic, and an inversion of the normally accepted hierarchical relationships in medicine, as indeed in anything else.

There is much which in a compendious piece has to be left unsaid. One must briefly refer to the energising and re-assessing effect that the new organic approach to medicine has had on Third World medicine. High technology medicine, essentially only available to a very few in such countries, is now perceived to represent a grotesque imbalance of resources. Instead, appropriate medical technology is proposed, and, for example, a debilitating disease such as diarrhoea in children is treated by the simplest oral rehydration technique; and, on another tack, a new Medical Building Design Unit has recently opened courses at the University of Bristol.

It is not surprising that so much has suddenly happened in the past very few years. The situation has been growing to the present climax since the late 1960s when Stewart Brand looked down on the revolving world from his Nebraska jet. It takes time, usually a generation, before the new becomes acceptable to the established ways of perception. We have now accomplished nearly 20 years of that period. We should therefore consider it highly probable that the once 'fringe' medicine, now 'alternative' medicine, will soon indeed become the 'complementary' medicine it seeks. The system it endeavours to complement is already capitulating.

Some problems remain. No one would expect or want medicine to yield up the rigour of scientific enquiry proper to its own field. No one would want complementary medicine to adopt those rigours for itself: the qualitative cost would be too great. Few would want complementary medicine to set up a system of qualifications and disciplinary bodies entirely analogous to that of the orthodox system. Their standards of expectation are not easily, if at all, quantifiable and the attempt to cut them to that Procrustean bed would reproduce the very impoverishment that the alternative system seeks to alleviate. A middle path to facilitate acceptance on both sides can be found. Each can pursue its own means while acknowledging the value of the other and incorporating such as is useful to it. It would be an enormous mistake to reduce the variety of species. Both should be part of the valid spectrum of medicine.

If one is foolhardy enough to speculate one would suppose that well before the end of the next ten years we shall see each side acknowledging the virtues of the other and agreeing to differ in their own perceptions and methods. The one will then be truly scientific both in name and attitude, and no longer conventional; the other will be, because it is accepted for all practical purposes within the pale of orthodox medicine, truly complementary.

It is cheering to suppose that by healing medicine we may also be helping to heal the wounds of an unusually aggressive, obsessive and sick society. By healing ourselves, we heal society and the medicine within it. But then, as the Persian proverb has it, 'if we truly seek the fountain of light, what use is the veil of words?'

